YOUR KNOWLEDGE HAS VALUE

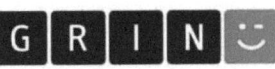

Latest Advancements, Application and Evolution of Biomaterials and Nanomaterials

Rangoli Srivastava

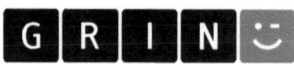

Bibliographic information published by the German National Library:

The German National Library lists this publication in the National Bibliography; detailed bibliographic data are available on the Internet at http://dnb.dnb.de.

ISBN: 9783389096789
This book is also available as an ebook.

© GRIN Publishing GmbH
Trappentreustraße 1
80339 München

Print and binding: Books on Demand GmbH, Norderstedt, Germany
Printed on acid-free paper from responsible sources.

The present work has been carefully prepared. Nevertheless, authors and publishers do not incur liability for the correctness of information, notes, links and advice as well as any printing errors.

GRIN web shop: https://www.grin.com/document/1524526

CONTENTS :

ABOUT THE AUTHOR

Dr.Rangoli Srivastava, currently working as an Assistant Professor in Department of Public Health Dentistry in Faculty of Dental Sciences, SGT University, Gurugram, Haryana. She is a dedicated public health dentist pursuing academic excellence in research related domains along with practicing dentistry.

Abstract

Several materials including biomaterials applied in varied aspects of Prosthodontics have demonstrated significant results since the advent of nanotechnology came into existence. Though, because the implementation of nanomaterials in prosthodontic s has tremendously improved several properties like modulus of elasticity, hardness of surface, polymerization shrinkage as well as loading property. Several nanocomposites made up of traditional metals or ceramics or resin etc. are now used extensively in prosthodontics. Most recent developments, technologies and advancements in terms of biomaterials and nanomaterials used in prosthodontics have been covered explicitly in this literature review. This review not only provides an extensive overview of the most recent pertinent discoveries, but it should also serve as a major impetus for additional study in terms of this topic. In prosthodontics, both biomaterials as well as nanomaterials have shown to be essential to the advancement of both fundamental research and operational technology. It illustrates how the numerous characteristics of prosthodontic materials, such as modulus of elastic modulus, the level of hardness of surface, shrinkage from polymerization, and filler loading, can all be significantly improved following the use of nanotechnology to reduce their scales from micrometer to nanometer size.

Keywords: Biomaterials, Nanomaterials, Biocompatibility, Osseointegration, Wear resistance, Bonding Strength

1. INTRODUCTION –

The integration of nanoparticles and biomaterials has led to revolutionary advances in prosthodontics in recent years. These developments have completely changed dental care by providing previously unheard-of increases in functionality, durability, and aesthetics. The inventive creation and use of biomaterials and nanotechnology has propelled tremendous progress in the prosthodontics sector. Thanks to their improved durability, biocompatibility, and aesthetic results, these materials have completely changed the way dental restorations are done. [1]

In the mid-1990s, the original author of this paper was a faculty member at Cornell University, where Richard P. Feynman's influence was still felt. Feynman, who taught at Cornell until 1951, had a profound influence on the university and the scientific community there. His "There's Plenty of Room at the Bottom" presentation at Caltech in December 1959 cemented his standing as a visionary and a trailblazer in the field of nanotechnology.

During his talk, Feynman covered a wide range of futuristic subjects, such as the manipulation of microscopic information, the possibility of developing sophisticated electron microscopes, the complexity of biological systems, the creation of small-scale computers, the difficulties of lubricating tiny scales, and the synthesis of materials and devices at the atomic and molecular levels. Even though he did not address dentistry in his speech, he demonstrated creative thinking in a television discussion with Murray Gell-Mann.

Feynman provided an example of how reevaluating commonplace activities, like brushing teeth, could result in original thoughts and discoveries. His capacity to stimulate and inspire thought in a variety of scientific fields is evidence of his ongoing influence and demonstrates that his legacy goes well beyond his roles and particular accomplishments.

Nanotechnology has come out of science fiction and into the real world since the time of Richard Feynman. Nowadays, a lot of Feynman's visions are a reality. These days, nanotechnology has a big influence on almost every field, including technology, science, and engineering. This trend is also present in the medical and dental disciplines. [2]

The unique qualities that nanomaterials and nanodevices exhibit—properties that were previously unattainable—are the reason for this extensive influence. These developments offer creative answers to problems that were previously deemed to be unsolvable.

In dentistry, nanotechnology is applied in many different ways. Among the subjects they address are dental materials, prosthodontics, endodontics, periodontics, implantology, regenerative dentistry, and diagnostic and restorative dentistry. Nanotechnology has allowed dental professionals to use entirely new instruments and equipment. For example, LED light curing units are now more effective and efficient because to nanotechnology. Additionally, dental hard tissues are shielded from acidic foods by nanotechnology, promoting tooth preservation. It is crucial for the progress and characterization of dental materials and hard tissues, among many other uses. These developments in nanotechnology have led to significant breakthroughs in both dentistry science and practice. [3]

A degree of subjectivity is often involved in the assessment of prosthodontic material qualities because dental research lacks standardized and well-defined evaluation standards. Despite these obstacles, the discipline of dentistry has experienced substantial breakthroughs and increased interest during the last five years. Many novel biomaterials have been introduced into dental practice as a result of this increase in interest.

Among these, zirconium-reinforced lithium silicate, yttria-stabilized zirconia (YTZP), titanium (Ti) and its alloys, and lithium-disilicate-reinforced glass ceramics are notable.

Acrylic resins that have better mechanical qualities have also gained popularity. Moreover, glass fibers and nanoparticles have a lot of potential as reinforcement for different resin architectures and base materials. The improvement of polymethyl methacrylate (PMMA) denture base materials by fillers and hybrid systems, which act as novel techniques of reinforcement, has been a noteworthy development. Although in vitro studies have historically accounted for the majority of research in this field, there is currently a rising need for in vivo investigations to gain a deeper understanding of the usefulness and performance of these materials in actual contexts. [4]

Its outstanding translucency and aesthetic characteristics have drawn attention to the recently created multicolored monolithic ceramic materials. These characteristics not only improve the materials' aesthetic appeal but also add to their exceptional longevity, which makes them perfect for applications requiring great strength. These ceramics are becoming a popular option in many dental and restorative procedures due to their strength and cosmetic advantages. Consequently, conservative therapies utilizing adhesively luted monolithic restorations have been adopted at a justifiable rate. [5]

These procedures are becoming more and more well-liked because they can produce aesthetically beautiful results without sacrificing structural integrity. The popularity of these cutting-edge materials highlights how well they may satisfy both practical and aesthetic requirements, highlighting how well-suited they are for a variety of dental applications.[6]

2. HISTORY -

One of the four classical Sanskrit writings from India composed between 3500 and 1800 BC is the Rig Veda, which tells the tale of a warrior queen by the name of Vishpla. When Vishpla's wounds healed, she was fitted with an iron prosthetic after losing her leg in combat. The use of sutures to treat cuts and lacerations is also mentioned in the book. The well-known Indian physician Sushruta penned a thorough treatise on a variety of ailments and surgical methods circa 600 BC. His rotating skin flap nasal repair technique is still in use today.

While linen sutures are said to have been used in Egypt 4000 years ago, sutures composed of vegetable fibers, leather, tendons, and horsehair were frequently utilized during the time of Sushruta. These prehistoric documents demonstrate humanity's persistent efforts to use extraneous materials—possibly the first biomaterials—to restore function to amputated limbs or organs. Until Dr. J. Lister introduced aseptic surgical techniques in the 1860s, internal implants frequently failed due to infection, despite the fact that exterior prosthetic devices had some success. Antibiotic discoveries in the middle of the 20th century considerably decreased surgical infections, which paved the way for the effective application of implants in a variety of medical sectors and significantly improved millions of people's quality of life.

Dental implants were quite popular in the past and demonstrated a great deal of progress. Iron dental implants were used, as evidenced by human remains from the first century AD found in a Gallo-Roman necropolis in France. Shell fragments used as a dental implant for a young woman from AD 600 were discovered in Honduras during an archaeological project in 1923. Skeletons from the Middle Ages have been discovered in the Middle East with ivory dental implants. With varying degrees of success, gold posts were first placed into tooth sockets after extraction in the early 1800s. This was followed by studies using metals like platinum. The Strock brothers in Boston tested Vitallium dental implants in the 1940s.

When Swedish researcher Ingvar Brånemark found in 1952 that titanium implants could effectively fuse with bone, it was a major breakthrough. These titanium implants are still in widespread use today, acting as anchors for dental crowns or prosthetics. [7,8]

Research at the nanoscale scale is not new, despite the appearance of nanotechnology. For millennia, the nanoscale range has been used in the study of biological systems and the manufacture of materials including colloidal dispersions, metallic quantum dots, and catalysts. For example, more than a millennium ago, the Chinese applied gold nanoparticles as an inorganic dye to give their porcelains a red hue.

Even though Faraday created a stable colloidal gold dispersion in 1857 that lasted nearly a century before being destroyed during World War II, the thorough research of colloidal gold didn't start until the middle of the 19th century. Because of its ability to interact with spinal fluids, colloidal gold has also been used medicinally to cure arthritis and identify illnesses.

5

Our ability to visualize, engineer, and work with systems at the nanoscale has improved recently. Modern nanotechnology is innovative because it combines a better understanding of atomic interactions with our ability to visualize and manipulate materials at this scale.

While the study of materials at the nanoscale has a long history, the present wave of nanotechnology is partially propelled by the semiconductor industry's efforts to miniaturize devices, which is bolstered by developments in nanometer-level characterisation and manipulation techniques. Moore's law, which predicts that gadget dimensions will halve roughly every 18 months, is followed by this pattern. In sharp contrast to the centimeter-scale contact transistor developed by Bardeen, Brattain, and Shockley in 1947, modern transistors are now found in the nanometer range.

Currently, a large number of scientists are investigating molecular and nanoscale electronics, which are built from single molecules or molecular monolayers. Despite the fact that existing devices function below the fundamental boundaries set by thermodynamics and quantum mechanics, limitations in the physics of the devices and materials have created hurdles in transistor design. For example, when devices scale, MOSFET off-currents grow exponentially, and problems such as power dissipation and chip overheating prevent further downsizing. Fundamental material constraints, such as the expansion of semiconductor band gaps when materials approach de Broglie's wavelength, will eventually prevent transistors from getting any smaller.

Miniaturization offers major breakthroughs that go beyond semiconductor-based electronics. Nanomedicine—the promising use of nanotechnology in medicine—is expanding quickly. The creation of tiny devices, sometimes referred to as nanorobots, for better therapy and diagnostics is a significant application in nanomedicine. [9]
Nanobots have enormous potential as drug delivery vehicles, disease early detection detectors, and possibly even as tools for the repair of genetic or metabolic abnormalities. Research on nanotechnology goes beyond just making gadgets smaller; materials with unusual physical characteristics at the nanoscale scale have been studied for a variety of uses.

For example, gold nanoparticles have several possible uses because of their consistent size and surface chemistry. By attaching different functional organic molecules or bio-components, they can function as adaptable carrier vehicles and enable varied capabilities.
Furthermore, bandgap-engineered quantum devices such as heterojunction bipolar transistors and lasers that display unique optical and electrical transport properties have been made possible by nanotechnology. The field of nanotechnology study has been further broadened by the introduction of synthetic materials such as carbon nanotubes, carbon fullerenes, and organized mesoporous materials. Characterization, measurement, and manipulation of nanostructures and nanomaterials have been transformed since the introduction of scanning tunneling microscopy (STM) in the early 1980s, and other scanning probe microscopy (SPM) techniques such as atomic force microscopy (AFM) have ensued since then. [10]

These technologies, when combined with existing techniques such as transmission electron microscopy (TEM), allow researchers to explore and modify nanostructures with remarkable atomic-level resolution. Although often invisible, nanotechnology is already present in many facets of our life. It symbolizes not only a novel technological advancement but also the amalgamation of current technologies with our recently acquired proficiency in seeing and modifying matter at the atomic level. Because of this, nanotechnology is attractive from a scientific, commercial, and political standpoint.[11]

3. APPROACHES OF NANOMATERIALS

Top-down and bottom-up approaches are the two main ways to synthesize nanomaterials and build nanostructures. When using a top-down technique, like attrition or milling, bigger materials are reduced to produce nanoparticles. On the other hand, the bottom-up method—which uses colloidal dispersion as an example—involves creating nanoparticles from atomic or molecule components. Lithography is a hybrid process that combines top-down etching and bottom-up thin-film growth, whereas nanolithography and nanomanipulation are more bottom-up approaches. Both strategies, each with pros and cons of its own, are essential to nanotechnology and play significant roles in contemporary business.

The top-down approach's main problem is surface imperfection. Traditional methods such as lithography have the ability to cause considerable harm to the crystal structure during the processing phase, even during the etching stages. For example, lithography-produced nanowires may have imperfections in their structure and frequently have uneven surfaces. Because of their high surface-to-volume ratio, these flaws have a significant impact on the surface chemistry and physical characteristics of nanostructures and nanomaterials. Surface flaws can decrease conductivity, which increases the risk of heat generation and complicates the design and construction of devices. Top-down methods are still essential for creating nanostructure and nanomaterials, despite these disadvantages.[12]

Although it is stressed in the literature on nanotechnology, the bottom-up method is not a novel idea in the synthesis of materials. By assembling components atom by atom or molecule by molecule, this process frequently produces structures with fewer flaws, a more uniform chemical composition, and improved ordering. While individual monomers are joined to form polymers in organic chemistry and polymer science, growth species unite to form crystal structures on a surface during crystal growth. When creating and working with nanostructures and nanomaterials, bottom-up techniques are essential, particularly when working with nanoscale dimensions. Bottom-up methods produce materials that are closer to thermodynamic equilibrium by minimizing internal stress and surface imperfections, in contrast to top-down methods.

Bottom-up methods are crucial in nanotechnology because they produce nanostructures with higher characteristics and performance.

4. APPLICATION OF NANOMATERIALS IN PROSTHODONTICS [13]

The field of prosthodontics, which focuses on making and fitting artificial replacements for teeth and other elements of the mouth, is using nanomaterials more and more. The following are some important applications of nanomaterials in this field:

1. Improved Dental Implants - Nanocoatings: By coating dental implants with nanomaterials, osseointegration—

the implants' integration with the jawbone—is improved. Titanium dioxide (TiO2) nanoparticles, for instance, have the ability to improve bone cell development and adhesion.

- Surface Modifications: The increased surface area of implants featuring nanostructured surfaces facilitates a quicker and more robust bonding process with bone tissue.

2. Better Dental Materials - Nanocomposites: Dental composites that contain silica and zirconia nanoparticles exhibit superior strength, resistance to wear, and visual appeal. Additionally, they are simpler to handle and polish.

- Nanofillers: By improving the mechanical qualities of dental resins and lowering shrinkage during polymerization, nanofillers help dental restorations last longer.

3. Antibacterial Properties - Nanoparticles: The antibacterial properties of silver nanoparticles are well-known. By adding these agents to dental materials, the risk of infection is reduced by inhibiting the growth of bacteria and the creation of biofilms.

- Nanostructured Coatings: By keeping germs from adhering to and proliferating on dental prosthesis, these coatings contribute to good oral hygiene and the avoidance of conditions like peri-implantitis.

4. Sturdier Denture Bases: Denture bases strengthened with nanofibers have a longer lifespan. For example, the incorporation of nanofibers into denture bases made of polymethyl methacrylate (PMMA) enhances their fracture resistance.

- Nanoclays: The mechanical qualities and stability of denture base materials are improved by the addition of nanoclays.

5. Advanced Tissue Engineering - Nanoscaffolds: To facilitate the growth and differentiation of cells required for the regeneration or repair of oral tissues, nanomaterials can be employed to produce scaffolds for tissue engineering.

- Growth Factors: By delivering growth factors in a regulated manner, nanoparticles can support the regeneration of soft tissues and bone surrounding dental implants.

6. Examining Instruments

- Nanosensors: Added to dental prostheses, nanosensors can track the condition of the tissues around them and identify early indicators of infection or implant failure.

- Nanobiosensors: These can monitor biochemical markers in real time, which helps with oral health management and treatment outcomes.

7. Enhancements in Appearance

- Nanoceramics: Because of their exceptional color-matching and translucency, veneers, crowns, and bridges composed of nanoceramic materials offer more aesthetic appeal.

- Nanopigments: These make it possible for dental restorations to precisely match color, ensuring that prosthesis seem natural in the mouth.

The use of nanomaterials in prosthodontics has greatly improved dental prosthesis' usability, robustness, and attractiveness. Nanotechnology has a major impact on prosthodontic treatments, leading to better patient outcomes through enhanced dental materials and improved implant integration and performance.

4.1 NANOIMPRESSION MATERIALS :

With the help of nanomaterials, imprint materials can be customized to meet certain requirements. An innovative siloxane impression medium incorporates nanofillers to improve precision. This invention has a number of benefits:

- Improved flow properties.
- Improved hydrophilic qualities lead to a decrease in the occurrence of voids, and impression accuracy is increased. [14]

4.2 NANOMETALS

Alloys based on cobalt are typically used to create metal frames for detachable partial dentures. When compared to conventional stainless steel and gold alloys, cobalt chromium molybdenum alloy, which evolved from its simpler binary alloy forms, has proven to offer greater mechanical strength and corrosion resistance.

Even with titanium's inherent benefits—specific strength, resistance to corrosion, biocompatibility, and elastic modulus—surface modification is essential to the long-term viability of titanium implants. Titanium nanoparticles have been investigated by researchers as a potential means of improving biological integration. By experimenting with anodic oxidation, Dorkhan and associates were able to create nanoscale pores in the 50 nm range on the surface of titanium implants. Soft-tissue cells including fibroblasts and keratinocytes adhered to both changed and unmodified implant surfaces similarly, according to their research. On the nanostructured surface, however, the adhesion of oral streptococci was greatly decreased.

Numerous studies have demonstrated that the straightforward and affordable technique of anodization can enhance osteoblastic adhesion. In order to demonstrate this, Yao and his colleagues used anodization to create nanostructured surfaces on titanium and Ti6Al4V implants in 2015. When compared to unanodized titanium-based surfaces, the modified surfaces showed more nanoscale roughness, which improved osteoblastic adhesion on the anodized metal substrates.[15]

4.3 NANOCERAMICS

Although widely used alumina ceramics have good mechanical qualities, one major disadvantage is that they are easily cracked. While zirconia ceramics have addressed some of these problems, they are not very durable. Ceramic materials with nanoscale dimensions in their microstructure phase are referred to as "nanoceramics". One of the main drawbacks of ceramics is their intrinsic brittleness; nevertheless, because of the arrangement of atoms at the nanoceramic interface, nanoceramics show increased toughness and ductility. Numerous research works have examined the strength and toughness of nanoceramics. In a study by Wang et al. (2006), for instance, nanoceramics outperformed a composite of AL203 and conventional ZrO2 when 20% Nano ZrO2 was added. According to Li et al. (2011), nano ZrO2 had a hardness of 1750 V, compared to 1500 for standard ZrO2.

In a similar vein, Raj et al. (2014) examined the microhardness and toughness of nano TiO2 ceramics against standard TiO2 ceramics, finding that nano TiO2 had greater hardness. In conclusion, extreme plasticity and better mechanical qualities are just two of the many benefits that come with using nanoceramics.[16]

4.4 NANORESINS

High hardness and stiffness are among the advantageous mechanical attributes of Poly Methyl Meth-Acrylate (PMMA), which are combined with enhanced biologic qualities including biocompatibility and attractiveness. It is also renowned for being simple to process. PMMA does, however, have a number of disadvantages, such as color instability, low resilience to wear and dimensional shrinkage, irritation of the oral mucosa, and discoloration. In addition, it has poor resistance to abrasion, low fatigue strength, and microbial adherence.

Numerous improved qualities are introduced when PMMA and nanoparticles are combined. To improve PMMA material, nanoparticles such as TiO2, ZrO2, and Carbon Microfiber Tubes (CMT) have been used. A study by Hua et al. (2013) evaluated the reinforcing power of TiO2-reinforced PMMA to regular PMMA. The results showed that the concentration of the strengthening reaction may be almost reached by nanoparticles with a ratio of aspect greater than thirty. A 3% volume grow, or a 6% volume boost in glass fiber, was also when saturation happened.[17]

A little amount of carbon nanotubes (CNT) added to PMMA greatly increases its impact strength, as Cooper et al. (2002) found. Tensile strength and modulus were increased when Methacryloxy-PropyltrimethoxySilane (MPS) modified silica nanoparticles were added to PMMA by Hong et al. (2003). The effects of adding different percentages of modified ZrO2 to heat-activated PMMA were studied by Mudhaffar (2012). Significant improvements were observed in fatigue resistance, tensile strength, and abrasion resistance, especially at 3% and 5% nanofiller concentrations.

Yoshida et al. (1999) showed the resin composite incorporating silver nanoparticles' persistent inhibitory action against the S. mutans bacterium in an effort to better understand the antibacterial capabilities of nanoparticles. PMMA composites containing additional TiO2 and Fe3O2 nanomaterials were developed by Laura et al. (2011) to improve their antibacterial properties and visual appeal. According to their findings, PMMA-containing nanoparticles showed decreased porosity and less Candida albicans cell adherence when compared to reference samples.[18]

4.5 NANOMATERIALS IN MAXILLOFACIAL MATERIALS

By covering silicone, Meran et al. (2017) carried out an in-vitro study to evaluate the efficacy of metallic nanoparticles against Candida albicans. In this investigation, human fibroblasts were used. They discovered that the application of a silver nanoparticle coating effectively stopped the growth of fungi, as shown by the decreased ethanol production by the yeast, with no endangering the fibroblasts in a cytotoxic way. The effects of incorporating titanium oxide (TiO2) nanofillers on the physical characteristics of room-temperature vulcanized (RTV) VST50F and high-temperature vulcanized (HTV) Cosmesil M511 maxillofacial silicone elastomers were investigated by Shakir DA et al. (2018) in a different study.

The findings demonstrated a statistically significant improvement in the materials' tear resistance, tensile force, elongation percentage, and hardness after 0.25 weight percent and 0.2 weight percent TiO_2 nanofillers were added to VST50F and Cosmesil M511 elastic materials, respectively.[19]

5. RECENT ADVANCES IN NANOMATERIALS

Recent developments in nanomaterials have had a significant impact on dentistry, offering improved alternatives for a range of dental materials and procedures. These are some significant recent advancements:

1. Enhanced Nanocomposites-Sturdiness and Strength: Modern dental composites are strengthened with nanoparticles such as zirconia, silica, and nanohydroxyapatite, which improves their mechanical characteristics and lengthens their lifespan.
- Minimized Shrinkage: Advances in nanocomposite formulations are designed to reduce gaps and minimize polymerization shrinkage, which enhances the fit and longevity of dental restorations.

2. Antibacterial Nanomaterials - Silver Nanoparticles: Adding silver nanoparticles to dental materials has demonstrated robust antimicrobial properties, which aid in inhibiting the growth of biofilms and bacterial colonization on dental surfaces.
- Copper and zinc nanomaterials: Due to their antibacterial qualities, these microscopic particles are also being investigated to serve as substitutes for silver nanoparticles in the treatment of oral infections.

3. The use of nanotechnology in Implants for Dentistry - Surface Nanostructuring: By encouraging improved bone cell adhesion and faster integration with the jawbone, nanostructured substances surfaces on dental implants improve osseointegration and consequently increase implant stability and durability.
- Drug-Delivering Nanocoatings: By delivering antibiotics or anti-inflammatory medications locally, novel nanocoatings on implants can lower the risk of surgical site infections and promote recovery.

4. Fluoride Nanoparticles: Thanks to advancements in nanotechnology, fluoride nanoparticles provide a more effective way to remineralize dental enamel than conventional fluoride treatments.
- Toothpaste containing nanohydroxyapatite particles: This non-fluoride alternative to toothpaste helps restore enamel's mineral content.

5. Tissue Science and Restorative Dentistry - Nanofiber Scaffolds: By offering the perfect conditions for cell development and differentiation, advances in nanofiber substrate technology enable tissue engineering, which helps to regenerate bone and periodontal tissues.
- Growth Factor Distribution: To encourage the regeneration of the jawbone and connective tissue surrounding dental implants, growth factors are delivered in a regulated manner using nanoparticles.

6. Better Dental Adhesives - Nanofillers that are in Adhesives: Adding nanofillers to dental adhesives increases their resistance to wear, durability, and bonding strength, which results in dental restorations that last longer.
- Nanoparticles for Desensitization: By occluring dentinal tubules, novel adhesive formulations including nanoparticles can lessen tooth sensitivity and improve patient comfort.

7. Aesthetic Enhancements - Nanoceramics: Because of their exceptional translucency and color-matching abilities, nanoceramics provide better aesthetics when used in dental restorations like veneers and crowns.

11

- Nanopigments: These let dental restorations match colors precisely, allowing prosthesis to look natural next to natural teeth.

Significant progress is being made in dentistry thanks to the use of nanomaterials, which improve both the functionality and appearance of dental procedures. These developments are improving the efficacy and durability of dental materials, encouraging better dental hygiene, and giving patients more consistent and visually beautiful results. It is anticipated that as research advances, nanotechnology will have many more applications in dentistry, providing even more cutting-edge dental care options.[20-24]

6. OUTCOME OF USING NANOMATERIALS

Significant progress is being made in dentistry thanks to the use of nanomaterials, which improve both the functionality and appearance of dental procedures. These developments are improving the efficacy and durability of dental materials, encouraging better dental hygiene, and giving patients more consistent and visually beautiful results. It is anticipated that as research advances, nanotechnology will have many more applications in dentistry, providing even more cutting-edge dental care options.

A relatively new field called nanodentistry has been impacted by the slow but steady introduction of nanotechnology into the dentistry industry. The utilization of nanomaterials, nanobiotechnology, nanorobots, and tissue engineering is anticipated to make it easier to restore and sustain the best possible oral health with nanodental technology. There is hope for both disease prevention and treatment through a variety of nanodentistry approaches, which will be covered in more detail in the sections that follow.[25]

7. OTHER APPLICATIONS OF NANOMATERIALS IN DENTISTRY

Apart from the above mentioned applications, nanomaterials are being used into dentistry to develop sophisticated diagnostic instruments such as small sensors and tiny biosensors, which have the ability to recognize precocious indications of dental disorders and continuously monitor oral health. They are lessening enamel degradation and increasing the efficacy of whitening treatments. Additionally, dental cements and sealants are becoming better because to nanotechnology, which enhances their adherence, strength, and longevity. One novel use involves the use of miniature diamonds in root canal therapy, which help to promote healing and sanitize the canals. These numerous uses demonstrate the enormous potential of nanoparticles to revolutionize several facets of dental care.[26]

8. INTRODUCTION TO BIOMATERIALS

Biomaterials are materials designed to interact with biological systems for therapeutic or diagnostic purposes in medicine. They are essential to contemporary medicine, especially in the area of prosthetics, where they are utilized to replace or support body parts that are ill or damaged. These materials, which can be synthetic or natural, are made to be biocompatible, which means that when they are implanted in the body, they won't cause an immunological reaction.

Biomaterials in Prosthodontics

Biomaterials are crucial to the prosthodontic field because they enable the creation of dental implants. Dental implants are an advanced use of biomaterials designed to replace lost teeth and improve the dentition's appearance and functionality. Dental implants have become increasingly popular over the last forty years, changing the sector with their cutting-edge designs and materials that provide predictable and long-lasting outcomes.[51]

Dental Implants: An Overview

Since their invention, dental implants have seen significant development. Modern implants are currently accepted as the gold-plated standard for tooth replacement, despite their early difficulties. A dental implant system's main job is to replicate the role of a normal tooth by transferring masticatory stresses to the mandibular or maxillary bone. To guarantee the long-term reliability and efficacy of the implant, it is essential to comprehend the spatial distribution of pressures and distortions inside the implant alongside the surrounding bone.

Crucial Elements of Implant Success

1. Bone Remodeling: In reaction to occlusal stresses and the formation of normal peri-implant soft tissue dimensions, bone remodeling takes place during the first year of function. The remodeling process may be either beneficial or detrimental, contingent upon the internal stress conditions brought about by the occlusal forces.

2. Osseointegration: The process by which an implant directly establishes a structural and functional relationship with living bone is called osseointegration, and it is a crucial component of implant success. The stability and lifespan of the implant are guaranteed by proper osseointegration.

3. Load Transfer: It's critical to understand how mechanical stresses are moved across an implant to the nearby bone. While high loading can result in component failure, improper load transfer can induce bone loss.

4. Design Parameters: An implant's design affects both its initial stability and long-term success. The implant's form, diameter, length, and surface properties are important design factors. The ability of the implant to fuse with the bone and endure functional stresses is influenced by each of these elements.

5. Healing and Loading: In order to prevent fibrous tissue encapsulation rather than osseointegration, it is crucial to avoid overloading during the early healing phase after implant placement. Bone structure and other individual characteristics determine the ideal time for healing prior to functional loading.

Implant Success Criteria

Certain standards were put forth by Albrektsson et al. to assess implant success:

1. In clinical settings, implants have to remain stationary.

2. A radiographic examination should reveal no peri-implant radiolucency.

3. After the first year of function, radiographic vertical bone loss should be less than 0.2 mm yearly.

4. Implants need to be free of discomfort, neuropathies, infections, and other issues.

5. After five years and ten years of observation, the success rate need to be at least 85% and 80%, respectively.

Obstacles and Things to Think About

Although these standards offer a foundation for analyzing implants, determining the success of a single implant can be difficult. Patients can have greatly different bone remodeling depending on occlusal stresses and bone quality, among other things. The risk of pressure necrosis or disuse atrophy emphasizes how crucial it is to carefully plan functional occlusal loads in order to preserve osseointegration and avoid implant failure.

In conclusion, sophisticated biomaterials, exact design specifications, and a comprehensive comprehension of bone-implant interactions are critical to the development and effective application of dental implants in prosthodontics. Dental implants will probably get even more dependable and efficient as science and technology advance, providing better results for people who are missing teeth.[52-55]

9. APPLICATION OF DIFFERENT TYPES OF BIOMATERIALS IN PROSTHODONTICS –

Dental Bioceramics

Bioceramics have come a long way from being inert implants to substances that actively interact with living tissues since they were first used before the 1970s. At first, bioceramics were mostly employed as passive tissue substitutes due to their physical characteristics. But the needs for bioceramics changed as our knowledge of the metabolic and regulatory processes of the human body expanded. In addition to their physical functions, modern bioceramics are projected to support tissue regeneration and improve quality of life. The promise of nanobioceramics, which promote tissue regeneration and healing and restore physiological functions, has been the driving force behind this change. [56]

When utilizing biomaterials, biocompatibility and functioning are the two main factors to take into account. Bioceramics also need to maintain their shape when subjected to physiological loads. The mechanical characteristics of ceramic components, particularly their strength, are essential for guaranteeing their safety and efficacy. Improving ceramics' mechanical strength is crucial since it affects all other qualities.

When compared to metals, bioceramics often have a lesser fracture toughness despite their hardness. Because of their ability to absorb energy and prevent crack propagation, metals have high toughness due to their crack-tip plasticity. Conversely, ceramics such as alumina show very little flexibility at the crack tips, which means that their energy absorption and fracture toughness are reduced. For instance, the fracture toughness (KIC) values of ductile metals like titanium alloys are roughly one-fiftieth that of ceramics like alumina.

An important breakthrough came with the advent of ceramics for orthopedic and maxillofacial implants in the early 1970s. Medical-grade bioceramics are made to be bioinert, which means they will remain stable in the human body for more than a decade. Impurity-free high-purity oxide ceramics are essential for preventing biological deterioration. The capacity of bioceramics to operate in the physiological environment without deforming and their biocompatibility are key factors in their success. Because of the significance of the interaction at the nanoscale bone/implant interface, surface alterations and micro- and nanoscale coatings have attracted attention as ways to improve these interactions. Nowadays, businesses are selling implants that have been altered at the nanoscale for use in maxillofacial, orthopedic, and dental procedures.

Physical Characteristics: Bioceramics' distinct mechanical, physical, and thermal characteristics enable a wide range of applications. Biocompatibility, strength, density, and wear resistance are critical in biomedical settings. Two important physical characteristics are density and porosity; open porosity can lower ceramic strength and enable liquid or gas access, which can influence performance.[57]

Bioceramics are classified according to the way their bodies react to them:

- Bioinert Ceramics: These materials do not cause a biological reaction; examples include zirconia ($ZrO2$) and alumina ($Al2O3$).

- Bioactive Ceramics: Glass ceramics and bioglass are two examples that bind to bone.

- Bioresorbable Ceramics: These include ceramics made of calcium phosphate, which break down and are eventually replaced by real bone.

Dental implants, maxillofacial surgery, and orthopedics all make substantial use of these materials. Ongoing advancements seek to increase performance and dependability while broadening their applications.

The processes utilized in the synthesis and production of bioceramics have a significant impact on their characteristics, uses, and physiological effects. In order to develop bioceramics that more effectively integrate with biological tissues and encourage healing and regeneration, current research is concentrated on advancing these techniques. Particularly exciting developments in surface engineering and nanotechnology present fresh chances to create sophisticated bioceramic materials. Bioceramics are dynamic substances that continuously interact with biological tissues, a far cry from their initial state as inert tissue substitutes. Their uses in prosthodontics and other medical specialties are still growing, thanks to developments in material science and a better comprehension of human physiology. Bioceramics's potential to promote and accelerate the body's natural healing processes will determine its future, ultimately leading to better patient outcomes and a higher standard of living.

10. NANOBIOCERAMICS AND NANOCOMPOSITES[59]

Materials that range in size from 1 to 100 nanometers are referred to as "nanostructured materials." Nanotechnology has been the driving force behind major breakthroughs in materials science and engineering during the past ten years. Because these materials are compatible with naturally occurring biological systems that display nanostructures, like protein complexes, viruses, and membranes, they hold great promise for usage in biomedical applications. Among the nanostructured materials that interact with the body, nanobioceramics is a promising class. By assisting the body's natural healing processes, they promote tissue regeneration and aid in the restoration of physiological functioning. The objective is to create a new class of nanobioceramics with more extensive medical uses.

Because porous materials allow natural bone to grow into the graft and form a strong link with the bone, they are becoming an increasingly popular choice for bone grafting. The effectiveness of bone grafts in medical procedures depends on this integration.

Mixtures with at least one nanoscale component are called nanocomposites. At this scale, it is possible to increase the mechanical characteristics of the composite, such as strength and stiffness, to make it more like genuine bone. The hydroxyapatite (HAp)-polymer composite is one such material that has rigidity similar to that of bone. By physically combining materials or adding new elements to already-existing nanostructured materials, nanocomposites can be created, which enables the alteration of properties and possible addition of new functions.

Another kind of nanocomposite that finds value in biomedical applications are gels, which are three-dimensional networks submerged in liquid. These gels can have nanostructured materials inserted in them to improve and customize their characteristics for certain biomedical applications. This technique makes it possible to precisely regulate the properties of the nanostructured elements inside the gel, which makes it easier to design specific biomedical devices. Numerous uses become possible when nanostructured materials are incorporated into biomedical equipment. They are perfect for a variety of medical applications because of their special qualities, which include promoting tissue regeneration and simulating the mechanical characteristics of real bone. The goal of the ongoing development of gel systems, nanocomposites, and nanobioceramics is to raise the efficiency and dependability of biomedical equipment.

The possibility of using nanobioceramics to encourage tissue regeneration is being investigated. These materials, which are especially helpful for orthopedics and dentistry, aid in the healing process and restore normal physiological functioning by interacting with the body's biological processes at the nanoscale. Because porous nanostructured materials can promote natural bone ingrowth, they are increasingly being used in bone grafting operations to provide a robust and long-lasting link between the graft and the host bone. This characteristic is critical to the long-term viability of implants and bone grafts, particularly in orthopaedic and maxillofacial surgery.

Customizing the mechanical characteristics of nanocomposites to closely resemble real bone is essential for developing materials that effectively interact with the body and support its activities. For example, hydroxyapatite-polymer composites have appropriate rigidity that imitates real bone, improving the functionality of implants and prosthetics. Nanostructured materials in gel systems open up new opportunities for biomedical applications. These gels can be designed to have particular qualities, which qualifies them for use in a variety of medical equipment. Highly specific and efficient biomedical solutions can be developed by adjusting the properties of the nanoparticles inside the gel. Innovations in nanostructured materials have had a big impact on the biomedical industry.

These materials have fascinating opportunities for medical applications, ranging from nanobioceramics that support tissue regeneration to nanocomposites that imitate the characteristics of genuine bone. It is anticipated that further research and development will increase the incorporation of nanostructured components into biomedical devices, resulting in better patient outcomes and novel therapeutic approaches.

11. CURRENT PRODUCTION TECHNIQUE

The characteristics and microstructure of ceramic materials
The manufacturing processes and production pathways of ceramic materials, such as bioceramics and nanoceramics, have a significant impact on their microstructure and properties. To give these materials the needed qualities, or a mix of desired attributes, the right synthesis process must be chosen.
Production Methods
Ceramic materials are often manufactured using pressing and wet chemical processing procedures including co-precipitation and sol-gel. Bio ceramics, tiny coatings, nanostructured solid forms, and nanoparticles are all made using these techniques.

In contemporary ceramics technology, pressing is the process of compacting powder by packing it into a mold and then applying pressure. For bioceramics, heat pressing and hot isostatic pressing are frequently employed. Higher densities and finer grain structures—which are necessary for bioceramics—are produced by hot isostatic pressing, which applies pressure and heat in all directions using a pressurized gas like argon or helium. On the other hand, hot pressing works better for making blocks, flat plates, and irregular parts.

Computer-Assisted Design and Manufacturing (CAD/CAM) -[60-65]

CAD/CAM technology, which was first used in dentistry in the 1970s and early 1980s, has drawn a lot of interest in the last thirty years. The accuracy and simplicity of creating dental structures and restorations are improved by this technique. CAD/CAM has three primary phases:

1. The acquisition of data by means of imaging technologies, including CT scans, which convert geometrical data into digital data.

2. Using computerized design programs to construct a three-dimensional model that incorporates the essential structures, such as abutments and crowns.

3. Utilizing a computer-assisted milling or polishing machine to produce the intended result. Prefabricated blocks consisting of different compositions and materials, like ceramics (like alumina and zirconia), resin materials, and metals (like titanium and its alloys) are commonly used as the beginning material.

Three-Dimensional (3D) Printing

The fabrication of complexly shaped ceramic components has undergone a revolution with the advent of 3D printing technology. 3D printing is being investigated for bioceramics, having first been developed for metals and polymers. Ceramics 3D printing is still in its infancy, but it should become more common.

Reduced manufacturing time and costs, less design restrictions, and enhanced surface polish and dimensional accuracy are some of the main benefits of 3D printing. This technique can also be used in conjunction with patient imaging technologies such as CT scans in dentistry and oral surgery.

Ceramics 3D printing is not without its difficulties, though. Material problems, like partial melting, require careful investigation. Furthermore, to optimize process settings and reduce residual thermal stress—which leads to cracks and crumbling in ceramic components—it is imperative to have a deeper understanding of the interaction between lasers and materials.

Post-Treatment Requirements[66]

Post-treatments are necessary for 3D-printed ceramic components made via selective laser sintering (SLS) or stereolithography, in contrast to metal and polymer components. In order to achieve the required mechanical and physical qualities, these treatments entail heat operations to sinter the powders and remove organic binders. Dimensional shrinkage can result from post-thermal treatments in an unanticipated way. A "staircase effect" may also appear on the surface as a result of the layer-by-layer building. By keeping each layer as thin as feasible, this can be reduced. Extra grinding or polishing procedures are required for surfaces with poor finishes. The minimum constituent element size of the printed item can be decreased by optimizing the raw materials, systems, and process parameters, which will enhance the surface finish and general quality.

Ceramic materials' characteristics and microstructure are closely related to the processes used in their manufacture. In order to create bioceramics and nanoceramics with desirable qualities, techniques like pressing, hot isostatic pressing, and wet chemical processing are essential. The precision and capacities of ceramic manufacturing are being improved by advanced technologies like CAD/CAM and 3D printing, but they still have issues that need more study and development. With ongoing advancements in material qualities and manufacturing techniques, ceramic materials appear to have a bright future in biomedical applications.

11.1 CALCIUM PHOSPHATE[70-73]

Because synthetic calcium phosphate closely resembles the natural hydroxyapatite present in bone in terms of both composition and structure, it is thought to be an ideal biomaterial for bone replacement. Despite its special qualities and reactivity in physiological contexts, the chemical properties of hydroxyapatite (HAp), a form of calcium phosphate, are usually assessed in the context of calcium phosphates.

It is well known that calcium phosphate is a biocompatible substance that chemically resembles the mineral elements of teeth and bone. But because it's brittle and inorganic, calcium phosphate's mechanical properties are very different from those of human bone, even though their composition is comparable. Unless changed, this restriction limits the use of porous hydroxyapatite in load-bearing applications.

Based on their solubility, ability to bind to surrounding tissues, and capacity to break down and be replaced by the development of new bone, calcium phosphates are classified. Calcium phosphate surface ions can interchange with those in the aqueous solution when exposed to biological fluids, and a variety of ions and molecules, including proteins and collagen, can adsorb onto the surface.

Applications in Dentistry and Medicine
Calcium phosphate bioceramics are osteoconductive, which means they promote bone formation and tissue ingrowth, even if they are not osteoinductive—that is, they cannot create bone when implanted in non-bone areas. Applications include maxillofacial reconstruction, bone space fillers, alveolar ridge augmentation, artificial eye and ocular implants, bone cement additives, ear implants, spine fusion, and implant coatings.

Compounds of Calcium Phosphorus
Among the different calcium phosphate compounds are:
- Dicalcium phosphate (DCP) - Amorphous calcium phosphate (ACP)
- TTCP, or tetracalcium phosphate
- Tricalcium Phosphate, which includes α- and β-TCP
- Calcium apatite (HAp)

Biocompatible Coatings and Synthetic Apatites -
The goal of early research on synthetic apatites was to comprehend the structure, composition, and characteristics of biological apatites, especially human enamel apatites. The manufacture and use of these materials in dentistry and medicine, especially their application as scaffolds for bone and tooth regeneration, have been the focus of research during the last thirty years.
α- and β-tricalcium phosphates, HAp, and biphasic calcium phosphate (a combination of β-tricalcium phosphate and HAp) are among the commercially accessible synthetic calcium phosphate biomaterials. Sometimes, biological sources including coral, marine algae, processed human bone, and bovine bone are used to create these materials.

11.2 Nanotechnology and Calcium Phosphate

Innovative techniques for producing artificial nanocoatings and calcium phosphate nanopowders that resemble bone have been made possible by nanotechnology. These nanoparticles provide new opportunities for the development of biocompatible implant coatings and extremely strong dental and orthopedic nanocomposites. Due to insufficient bioactivity, metal implants, such as titanium and its alloys, frequently experience loosening over time. Osteointegration is improved by calcium phosphate sol-gel crystalline nanocoatings on a variety of substrates, including titanium and cobalt-chromium alloys.[74]

Production Techniques and Challenges

There are several ways to create calcium phosphate nanopowders and nanoplatelets that resemble bone, but the sol-gel approach shows the most promise. Monophasic calcium phosphate powders and coatings are more difficult to synthesize than biphasic sol-gel HAp products, which are comparatively easy to make. Because of their large surface areas, calcium phosphate nanoparticles and nanoplatelets provide good bioactivity for bone incorporation.

Since synthetic calcium phosphate closely resembles the structure and content of natural hydroxyapatite, it is a useful biomaterial for replacing lost bone. Its biocompatibility and capacity to promote bone formation make it appropriate for a range of medical and dental applications, notwithstanding its mechanical limits. Technological developments in nanotechnology and industrial methods keep improving the integration and performance of biomaterials based on calcium phosphate.

11.3 ZIRCONIA

ZrO_2, also referred to as zirconia, is zirconium in its fully oxidized state. Depending on the temperature, it can exist in several phases. However, there are significant industrial problems that prevent the production of pure zirconia. Zirconia is usually stabilized during heat treatment to stop expansion mismatch cracks from forming. Because it keeps zirconia ceramics from breaking and cracking, this stability is essential.

The use of alumina as a biomaterial was followed by the usage of zirconia in the dental and other sectors. However, depending on the synthesis method and intended usage, the zirconia employed is typically partially stabilized zirconia (PSZ), which is a combination of zirconia with other compounds such yttria, calcia, or magnesium oxide.

As dental implants and abutments, zirconia—especially PSZ—has grown in popularity in implant dentistry. ZrC with a tiny amount of stabilizing chemicals is referred to as partially stabilized zirconia, or PSZ for short. PSZ-based ceramic materials have various advantages over alumina, including better flexural strength, fracture toughness, and resistance to corrosion, all of which help to stop crack propagation and catastrophic failure. Zirconia ceramics' crystalline structure has a significant impact on their mechanical qualities and endurance. Three distinct phases can be seen in zirconia: cubic, tetragonal, and monoclinic. Elevated temperatures cause a change of the tetragonal phase, which is responsible for zirconia's exceptional mechanical characteristics. At lower temperatures, these phase transitions are stabilized by metallic oxides such as yttria.

Medical applications frequently employ tetragonal zirconia polycrystals (TZP), a form of partially stabilized zirconia. In particular, yttria-stabilized TZP (Y-TZP) ceramics show the "transformation toughening" effect, in which compressive stress is created during phase transformation by volumetric expansion, preventing the onset and propagation of cracks. However, excessive metastability is less desired for medical implants because, in some cases, it might result in catastrophic outcomes. Therefore, zirconia's successful use in biomedical applications depends on maintaining the proper stability balance.[75,76]

11.4 ALUMINA

Alumina, or aluminum oxide, is a widely utilized material in ceramics, particularly in applications related to biomedicine (Al_2O_3). Due to the high melting temperature of alumina ceramics, high-temperature sintering is necessary during the manufacturing process. Utilizing the Bayer method, alumina powder is produced from bauxite as the basic material. Alumina is typically white, but depending on purity or additives like chromium oxide, it can also be pink or brown. The color of alumina hence varies.

Since the 1970s, alumina has been utilized in orthopedic and dental applications, with quality control standards established by multiple organizations. Small-grain microstructure in medical-grade alumina prevents fatigue and crack formation under load.

Additives such as magnesium oxide can be added during processing to enhance the density and microstructure. One disadvantage is that a fibrous membrane may form at the contact between the implant and bone, which could cause the implant to dislodge.

Alumina is fragile, yet it has good hardness, low wear rates, and resilience to corrosion, which makes it a good material for orthopedic articulating surfaces. Predictions of long-term survival indicate excellent dependability under physiological stressors. Applications for alumina can be found in femoral head components and dental implants, among other orthopedic and dental implants.

Another ceramic utilized in clinical applications is partially stabilized zirconia (PSZ), which has better toughness than alumina. Zirconia-toughened alumina, however, would result from combining the best qualities of both alumina and zirconia in a perfect material.

This new generation of ceramic has processes via which stress-induced transformation-toughening can improve strength and fracture toughness.

The improvement of mechanical qualities has been the focus of recent developments in zirconia-toughened alumina ceramics; nonetheless, comprehensive evaluation of their efficacy will require long-term clinical research. A novel zirconia-toughened alumina ceramic, for example, was created in 2002 and has promise; however, additional clinical research is needed to prove its applicability as a high-performance biomaterial. [77]

11.5 BIOACTIVE GLASS

Since its discovery in the 1960s, the field of bioactive glasses and glass ceramics has experienced substantial advancements. These materials, which were first developed by Hench and associates, have special qualities that make them excellent choices for a range of medical applications. For instance, Bioglass® has great machinability and quick setting time in addition to the capacity to form bonds with living tissues. The materials' composition and shape can be changed to modify these characteristics, which makes them adaptable for use in tissue engineering projects as well as orthopedic, maxillofacial, and dental procedures.

It has been discovered that silicon, an essential trace element in the human body, is critical for bone mineralization and growth. Research has demonstrated that dental pulp stem cells can develop more readily on silicon scaffolds, suggesting a possible use for these scaffolds in tissue engineering applications. Researchers have created a new family of bioactive calcium silicate ceramics with customized compositions that promote osteogenic differentiation and bone formation in vitro and in vivo, drawing inspiration from the physiological roles of silicon.[78]

Bioglass® 45S5, one of the first bioactive glasses, was created in 1971. Due to the quick surface exchange of alkali ions with hydronium ions, it has higher osteoblastic activity than hydroxyapatite. As a result of this exchange, a silica-rich layer gradually forms, which facilitates the migration and combination of phosphate and calcium ions from the solution to create an amorphous $CaO-P_2O_5$ layer. Comparable occurrences have been found in bioglasses with marginally altered compositions.

The capacity of alternative bioactive glasses in the $Na_2O-CaO-P_2O_5-SiO_2$ system to form bonds with bone has been investigated, in addition to Bioglass. On the other hand, difficulties like crystallization and phase separation may impact their bioactivity. [79]

A range of manufacturing processes, such as flame spray synthesis and sol-gel processing, have been utilized in addition to traditional glass melting to create bioactive glass nanoparticles and nanofibers with targeted characteristics.

Bioactive glass composites have been studied for biomedical applications such dental implants and bone regeneration. These composites combine the bioactive qualities of glass with the mechanical capabilities of metals or polymers. By improving characteristics like flexibility and load-bearing capacity, these composites may find greater use in medical contexts.

Bioactive glasses have showed potential for dental treatments, maxillofacial surgery, and bone augmentation in biomedical applications. Although their antibacterial properties might restrict their application in some circumstances, they have also been investigated for ear, nose, and throat procedures. All things considered, bioactive glasses are a promising class of materials for medical applications. Current research is concentrated on resolving issues like brittleness and production costs to allow for a wider usage of these materials in implants and medical devices.[80]

11.6 RECENT ADVANCES IN BIOMATERIALS[81-85]

Recent years have witnessed tremendous progress in the field of biomaterials, especially in the areas of tissue engineering and medical implants. Among the noteworthy innovations are the incorporation of chemicals derived from plants, novel bonding materials, and enhanced grafting methods. Here, we examine current developments in four main areas: dental bone transplants, pectins, bonding polymers, and titanium implant coatings derived from plant products.

Titanium implant coatings derived from plant products

Because of their mechanical qualities and biocompatibility, titanium implants are utilized extensively. However, by coating the titanium with compounds generated from plants, the contact between the implant surface and its biological surroundings can be further strengthened. The objectives of these coatings are to enhance osseointegration, lower the risk of infection, and quicken healing. For example, bioactive plant chemicals like flavonoids and polyphenols have been employed to make coatings that are osteoconductive and antibacterial. These organic substances demonstrate anti-inflammatory qualities as well as encouraging cell adhesion and proliferation, both of which are critical for the long-term viability of implants.

Pectins

Plant cell walls include complex polysaccharides called pectins, which are well-known for their biocompatibility and gelling abilities. Because pectins may produce hydrogels, which are useful for drug delivery systems and wound healing, they are being investigated for a variety of uses in the biomedical area. In order to improve pectins' mechanical qualities and rates of degradation, recent research has concentrated on changing their molecular weight and esterification level. Pectins can now be employed in scaffolds for tissue engineering, where they can promote tissue regeneration and cell proliferation.

Materials for Bonding

For implants and other medical equipment to operate better and last longer, new bonding materials must be developed. Bioactive glass and ceramics are recent inventions that interact favorably with biological tissues in addition to providing strong mechanical connections. These substances have the ability to release healing ions that promote bone regrowth. Furthermore, the application of nanotechnology has resulted in the development of nanocomposites with improved mechanical strength, regulated degradation rates, and higher adhesive qualities. These advancements are especially helpful in orthopedic and dental applications where bond stability and duration are crucial.

Dental Bone Transplants

In situations where there is tooth loss or periodontal disease, dental bone transplants are crucial for bone regeneration and healing. In order to improve bone grafting's efficacy and patient outcomes, recent advancements have concentrated on enhancing the materials and techniques employed. The introduction of artificial bone replacements, which are made to resemble natural bone, is one noteworthy advancement. These substances, which are progressively reabsorbed by the body, serve as a scaffold for the formation of new bone and are frequently made of bioactive glasses or calcium phosphates. Additionally, it has been demonstrated that using growth factors and stem cells with graft materials can speed up bone regeneration and enhance the quality of the bone that is produced.

Additional uses of biological materials in dentistry

In conclusion, the field of biomaterials is quickly developing, and new methods are being developed to improve the functionality and integration of medical implants and grafts. Innovative dental bone grafts, sophisticated pectins, plant-derived coatings, and state-of-the-art bonding materials are just a few of the fascinating advancements influencing the direction of biomedical engineering. These developments not only lead to better patient outcomes but also open the door to longer-lasting and more efficient medical interventions.

Beyond prosthodontics, biomaterials are important in many other dental specialties, including endodontics, periodontics, and orthodontics. Biomaterials are utilized in endodontics for root canal fills and sealing; bioactive glass and bioceramics offer improved sealing qualities and encourage periapical healing.

Biomaterials such as collagen membranes and bone grafts are used in periodontics to replace damaged soft tissues and bone surrounding teeth through directed tissue regeneration and periodontal regeneration.

Biomaterials are useful to orthodontics because they allow for the creation of brackets and aligners that are more aesthetically pleasing, more comfortable, and more effective in moving teeth. In order to prevent cavities and encourage the remineralization of enamel, bioactive chemicals and antimicrobial coatings are also being added to restorative materials. This will increase the longevity and health of dental restorations. These uses highlight the adaptability and significance of biomaterials in improving patient outcomes and dental treatment.

12. CONCLUSION

The area of prosthodontics has undergone a revolution in recent years due to the incorporation of biomaterials and nanomaterials, which has improved the usefulness, durability, and aesthetics of dental procedures in ways never seen before. Although unrelated to dentistry, Richard P. Feynman's groundbreaking discoveries in the field of nanotechnology set the stage for the revolutionary developments that we are seeing today. The history of dental implants, from prehistoric times to contemporary discoveries, is a reflection of humanity's never-ending search for novel ways to restore oral function and health. From science fiction to science fact, nanotechnology has advanced significantly across a number of dental specialties, not just prosthodontics. Applications in implantology, regenerative dentistry, periodontics, restorative dentistry, and preventative care demonstrate the broad significance of nanoparticles in dentistry.

Current developments in nanomaterials have further strengthened dental implants, dental materials, tissue engineering, and diagnostic tools, improving patient outcomes and laying the groundwork for future developments in even more sophisticated solutions. Dentistry is developing thanks to the use of nanomaterials; new therapies that maintain both function and aesthetic appeal are available, and this will ultimately change the face of oral healthcare.

New developments in biomaterials have led to creative solutions for a range of medicinal uses. Utilizing the biocompatibility and antibacterial qualities of natural materials, plant product-based coatings for titanium implants offer a novel approach to improving implant integration and lowering the risk of infection. Fruit and vegetable-derived pectins, with their tunable mechanical characteristics and biocompatibility, have emerged as promising biomaterials for tissue engineering. Additionally, advancements in bonding materials have produced stronger and more resilient interfaces between tissues and biomaterials, extending the useful life and functionality of medical implants.

New methods and materials are being investigated in the field of dental bone grafts to improve implant stability and bone regeneration, which could lead to improved results for people having dental work done. These latest developments highlight the biomaterials' continuous evolution and open the door to more adaptable and efficient medical treatments.

13. REFERENCES :

1. Sybil D. Anatomic challenges in surgical reconstruction and functional rehabilitation of maxillofacial skeleton. Int J Recent Sci Res. 2018;9(2):23899–903.

2. Booth PW, Schendel SA, Hausamen JE. Maxillofacial surgery, vol. 2. 2nd ed. Philadelphia, PA: Elsevier; 2007. p. 83–92.

3. Guerrero-Santos J, Altamirano JT. The use of lingual flaps in repair of fistulas of the hard palate. Plast Reconstr Surg. 1996;38:123–8.

4. Tiwari R. Masseter muscle crossover flap in primary closure of oral-pharyngeal defects. J Laryngol Otol. 1987;101:172–8.

5. Egyedi P. Utilization of the buccal fat pad for the closure of oro-antral and oro-nasal communications. J Maxillofac Surg. 1977;5:241–4.

6. Cohen IK, Edgerton MT. Transbuccal flaps for the reconstruction of the floor of mouth. Plast Reconstr Surg. 1971;48:8–10.

7. Lentz J. Ankylose osseuse de la mâchoire inférieure, résection du col condyle avec interposition du muscle temporal entre les surfaces de résection. Congrés Franc de Chir 1895;113.

8. McGregor IA. The temporal flap in intra-oral cancer. Br J Plast Surg. 1963;16:318–23.

9. McGregor IA, Jackson IT. The extended role of the deltopectoral flap. Br J Plast Surg. 1970;23:173–9.

10. Jiano J. Paralizie faciale dupa extriparea unei tumori a parotidee trata prin operatia dlui gomoue. Bull Mem Soc Clin Bucharest 1908:22.

11. Conley J. Use of composite flaps containing bone for major repairs in the head and neck. Plast Reconstr Surg. 1972;49:522–6.

12. Ariyan S. The pectoralis major myocutaneous flap: a versatile flap for reconstruction in the head and neck. Plast Reconstr Surg. 1979;63:73–81.

13. Futrell JW, Johns ME, Edgerton MT, et al. Platysma myocutaneous flap for intraoral reconstruction. Am J Surg. 1978;136:504–7.

14. Quillen CG, Shearing JG, Georgade NG. Use of Latissmusdorsimyocutanoeus island flap for reconstruction in the head and neck area: case report. Plast Reconstr Surg. 1978;62:113–7.

15. Martin D, Pascal JF, Baudet J, Mondie JM, Farhat JB, Athoum A, et al. The submental island flap: a new donor site: anatomy and clinical applications as a free or pedicled flap. Plast Reconstr Surg. 1993;92:867–73.

16. Wang HS, Shen JW, Ma D, Wang JD, Tian AL. The infrahyoidmyocutaneous flap for reconstruction after resection of head and neck cancer. Cancer. 1986;57:663–8.

17. Taylor GI. Reconstruction of mandible with free composite iliac bone grafts. Ann Plast Surg. 1982;9:361–8.

18. Ueba Y, Fujikawa S. Nine years follow up of a free vascularized fibular graft in neuro fibromatosis: a case report and literature review. Int J Orthop Trauma Surg. 1983;26:595–600.

19. O'Brien BM, Morrison WA. Reconstructive microsurgery, vol. 76. Edinburgh: Churchill Livingstone; 1987. p. 97–101.

20. Soutar DS, Scheker LR, Tanner NSB, McGregor IA. The radial forearm flap: a versatile method for intraoral reconstruction. Br J Plast Surg. 1983;36:1–8.

21. dos Santos LF. The vascular anatomy and dissection of the free scapular flap. Plast Reconstr Surg. 1984;73:599–605.

22. McCraw JB, Furlow LT. The dorsalis pedis arterialized flap. Plast Reconstr Surg. 1975;55:177–85.

23. Forrest C, Boyd JB, Manktelow RT, Zuker R, Bowen V. The free vascularized iliac crest tissue transfer: donor site complications associated with 82 cases. Br J Plast Surg. 1992;45:89–93.

24. Han Y, Kiat-amnuay S, Powers JM, Zhao Y. Effect of Nano-oxide concentration on the mechanical properties of a maxillofacial silicone elastomer. J Prosthet Dent. 2008;100:465–73.

25. Guttal SS, Patil NP, Nadiger RK, Hasti A. Nasal prosthesis for a patient with mammalian bite injury. Case report. J Indian Prosthodont Soc. 2007;7:43–5.

26. Guttal SS, Patil NP, Shetye AD. Case report: Prosthetic rehabilitation of a midfacial defect resulting from lethal midline granuloma—a clinical report. J Oral Rehabil. 2006;33:863–7.

27. Guttal SS, Patil NP, Nadiger RK, Rachana KB, Dharnendra, Basutkar N. Use of acrylic resin base as an aid in retaining silicone orbital prosthesis. J Indian Prosthodont Soc. 2008;8:112–5.

28. Avinash CKA, Nadiger R, Guttal SS, Lekha K. Orbital prosthesis: a novel treatment approach. Int J Prosthodont Restor Dent. 2012;2(1):19–23.

29. Guttal SS, Patil NP, Thakur S, Kumar SMV, Kulkarni S. Implant-retained nasal prosthesis for a patient following partial rhinectomy: a clinical report. J Prosthodont. 2009;18:353–8.

30. Guttal SS, Shanbhag S, Kulkarni SS, Thakur SL. Rehabilitation of a missing ear with an implant retained auricular prosthesis. J Indian Prosthodont Soc. 2015;15:70–5.

31. Guttal SS, Desai J, Kudva A, Patil BR. Rehabilitation of orbital defect with silicone orbital prosthesis retained by dental implants. Indian J Ophthalmol. 2016;64:93–5.

32. Melek LN. Tissue engineering in oral and maxillofacial reconstruction. Tanta Dent J. 2015;12(3):211–23.

33. Zayed SM, Alshimy AM, Fahmy AE. Effect of surface treated silicon dioxide nanoparticles on some mechanical properties of maxillofacial silicone elastomer. Int J Biomater. 2014;2014:750398, 7 p.

34. Van Schooneveld MM, Vucic E, Koole R, et al. Improved biocompatibility and pharmacokinetics of silica nanoparticles by means of a lipid coating: a multimodality investigation. Nano Lett. 2008;8(8):2517–25.

35. Shakir DA, Abdul-Ameer FM. Effect of nano-titanium oxide addition on some mechanical properties of silicone elastomers for maxillofacial prostheses. J Taibah Univ Med Sci. 2018;13(3):281–90.

36. Mitra A, Choudhary S, Garg H, et al. Maxillofacial prosthetic materials-an inclination towards silicones. J Clin Diagn Res. 2014;8(12):ZE08–13.

37. Alsmael MA, Moudhaffer M, Ali M, et al. The effect of nano titanium silicate addition on some properties of maxillofacial silicone material. J Res Med Dent Sci. 2018;6:127–32.

38. Salih SI, Oleiwi JK, Ali HM. Modification of silicone rubber by added PMMA and natural nanoparticle used for maxillofacial prosthesis applications. ARPN J Eng Appl Sci. 2019;14(4):781–91.

39. Yazdani J, Ahmadian E, Sharifi S, et al. A short view on nanohydroxyapatite as coating of dental implants. Biomed Pharmacother. 2018;105:553–7.

40. García C, Ceré S, Durán A. Bioactive coatings deposited on titanium alloys. J Non-Cryst

Solids. 2006;352(32–35):3488–95.

41. Breding K, Jimbo R, Hayashi M, et al. The effect of hydroxyapatite nanocrystals on osseointegration

of titanium implants: An in vivo rabbit study. Int J Dent. 2014;2014:171305.

42. Svanborg LM, Hoffman M, Andersson M, et al. The effect of hydroxyapatite nanocrystals

on early bone formation surrounding dental implants. Int J Oral Maxillofac Surg.

2011;40(3):308–15.

43. Carinci F, Lauritano D, Bignozzi CA, et al. A new strategy against peri-implantitis: antibacterial

internal coating. Int J Mol Sci. 2019;20(16):3897.

44. Romanò CL, Tsuchiya H, Morelli I, et al. Antibacterial coating of implants: are we missing

something? Bone Joint Res. 2019;8(5):199–206.

45. Wafa H, Grimer RJ, Reddy K, et al. Retrospective evaluation of the incidence of early periprosthetic

infection with silver-treated endoprostheses in high-risk patients: case-control

study. Bone Joint J. 2015;97-B(2):252–7.

46. Akash RN, Guttal SS. Effect of incorporation of nano-oxides on color stability of maxillofacial

silicone elastomer subjected to outdoor weathering. J Prosthodont. 2015;24:569–75.

47. Kiat-Amnuay S, Mekayarajjananonth T, Powers JM, Chambers MS, Lemon JC. Interactions

of pigments and opacifiers on color stability of MDX4–4210/type A maxillofacial elastomers

subjected to artificial aging. J Prosthet Dent. 2006;95:249–57.

48. Haug SP, Andres CJ, Moore BK. Color stability and colorant effect on maxillofacial elastomers.

Part III: weathering effect on color. J Prosthet Dent. 1999;81:431–8.

49. Polyzois GL. Color stability of facial silicone prosthetic polymers after outdoor weathering. J

Prosthet Dent. 1999;82:447–50.

50. Zardawi FM, Xiao K. Optimization of maxillofacial prosthesis. In: Prosthesis. London:

IntechOpen; 2019. https://doi.org/10.5772/intechopen.85034.

51. Petrovic V, Zivkovic P, Petrovic D, Stefanovic V. Craniofacial bone tissue engineering. Oral

Surg Oral Med Oral Pathol Oral Radiol. 2012;114(3):e1–9.

52. Genden EM. Reconstruction of the mandible and the maxilla: the evolution of surgical technique.

Arch Facial Plast Surg. 2010;12(2):87–90.

53. Leucht P, Kim J-B, Amasha R, James AW, Girod S, Helms JA. Embryonic origin and Hox status determine progenitor cell fate during adult bone regeneration. Development. 2008;135(17):2845–54.

54. Karaplis AC. Chapter 3—Embryonic development of bone and regulation of intramembranous and endochondral bone formation. In: Bilezikian JP, Raisz LG, Martin TJBT, editors. Principles of bone biology. 3rd ed. San Diego, CA: Academic Press; 2008. p. 53–84.

55. Peer LA. Fate of autogenous human bone grafts. Br J Plast Surg. 1951;3(4):233–43.

56. Sullivan WG, Szwajkun PR. Revascularization of cranial versus iliac crest bone grafts in the rat. Plast Reconstr Surg. 1991;87(6):1105–9.

57. Abzhanov A, Rodda SJ, McMahon AP, Tabin CJ. Regulation of skeletogenic differentiation in cranial dermal bone. Development. 2007;134(17):3133–44.

58. Ratner BD, Hoffman A, Schoen FJ, Lemons JE. Biomaterials science: an introduction to materials in medicine. 3rd ed. Kidlington, Oxford: Academic/Elsevier; 2012. p. 1–1555.

59. Kolk A, Handschel J, Drescher W, Rothamel D, Kloss F, Blessmann M, et al. Current trends and future perspectives of bone substitute materials—from space holders to innovative biomaterials. J Craniomaxillofac Surg. 2012;40(8):706–18.

60. Bhatt RA, Rozental TD. Bone graft substitutes. Hand Clin. 2012;28(4):457–68.

61. Jakoi AM, Iorio JA, Cahill PJ. Autologous bone graft harvesting: a review of grafts and surgical techniques. Musculoskelet Surg. 2015;99(3):171–8.

62. Griffin KS, Davis KM, McKinley TO, Anglen JO, Chu TMG, Boerckel JD, et al. Evolution of bone grafting: bone grafts and tissue engineering strategies for vascularized bone regeneration. In: Clinical reviews in bone and mineral metabolism, vol. 13. Totowa, NJ: Humana Press Inc.; 2015. p. 232–44.

63. Statement of the American Association of Tissue Banks. 2009. Available from: https://www.aatb.org/.

64. Schlegel AK, Donath K. BIO-OSS—a resorbable bone substitute? J Long-Term Eff Med Implants. 1998;8(3–4):201–9.

65. Rombouts C, Jeanneau C, Camilleri J, Laurent P, About I. Characterization and angiogenic potential of xenogeneic bone grafting materials: role of periodontal ligament cells. Dent Mater J. 2016;35(6):900–7.

66. White E, Shors EC. Biomaterial aspects of Interpore-200 porous hydroxyapatite. Dent Clin N Am. 1986;30(1):49–67.

67. Shors EC. Coralline bone graft substitutes. Orthop Clin North Am. 1999;30(4):599–613.

68. Oryan A, Alidadi S, Moshiri A, Maffulli N. Bone regenerative medicine: classic options, novel strategies, and future directions. J Orthop Surg Res. 2014;9:1–27.

69. Ghassemi T, Shahroodi A, Ebrahimzadeh MH, Mousavian A, Movaffagh J, Moradi A. Current concepts in scaffolding for bone tissue engineering. Arch Bone Joint Surg. 2018;6(2):90–9.

70. Pei M, Li JT, Shoukry M, Zhang Y. A review of decellularized stem cell matrix: a novel cell expansion system for cartilage tissue engineering. Eur Cell Mater. 2011;22:333–43.

71. Song R, Murphy M, Li C, Ting K, Soo C, Zheng Z. Current development of biodegradable polymeric materials for biomedical applications. In: Drug design, development and therapy, vol. 12. Albany, NY: Dove Medical Press Ltd.; 2018. p. 3117–45.

72. Zheng YF, Gu XN, Witte F. Biodegradable metals. Mater Sci Eng R Rep. 2014;77:1–34.

73. Kamrani S, Fleck C. Biodegradable magnesium alloys as temporary orthopaedic implants: a review. Biometals. 2019;32(2):185–93.

74. Sidambe AT. Biocompatibility of advanced manufactured titanium implants—a review. Materials. 2014;7(12):8168–88.

75. Niinomi M, Nakai M. Titanium-based biomaterials for preventing stress shielding between implant devices and bone. Int J Biomater. 2011;2011:836587.

76. Takizawa T, Nakayama N, Haniu H, Aoki K, Okamoto M, Nomura H, et al. Titanium fiber plates for bone tissue repair. Adv Mater. 2018;30(4):1703608.

77. Li Y, Yang C, Zhao H, Qu S, Li X, Li Y. New developments of Ti-based alloys for biomedical applications. Materials. 2014;7(3):1709–800.

78. Rodriguez IA, Selders GS, Fetz AE, Gehrmann CJ, Stein SH, et al. Barrier membranes for dental applications: a review and sweet advancement in membrane developments. Mouth Teeth. 2018;2(1):1–9.

79. Cohen R. A porous tantalum trabecular metal: basic science. Am J Orthop (Belle Mead NJ). 2002;31(4):216–7.

80. Clinical evidence reveals unique biological response to Trabecular Metal dental implant. Available from: https://us.dental-tribune.com/news/clinical-evidence-reveals-unique-biologicalresponse-to-trabecular-metal-dental-implant/.

81. Yang K, Ren Y. Nickel-free austenitic stainless steels for medical applications. Sci Technol Adv Mater. 2010;11(1):14105.

82. Zhou FY, Qiu KJ, Bian D, Zheng YF, Lin JP. A Comparative in vitro Study on Biomedical Zr–2.5X (X = Nb, Sn) Alloys. J Mater Sci Technol. 2014;30(4):299–306.

83. Zhang Q, Wu W, Qian C, Xiao W, Zhu H, Guo J, et al. Advanced biomaterials for repairing and reconstruction of mandibular defects. Mater Sci Eng C. 2019;103:109858.

84. Bonda DJ, Manjila S, Selman WR, Dean D. The Recent Revolution in the Design and Manufacture of Cranial Implants: Modern Advancements and Future Directions. Neurosurgery. 2015;77(5):814–824. https://doi.org/10.1227/NEU.0000000000000899.

85. Cionca N, Hashim D, Mombelli A. Zirconia dental implants: where are we now, and where are we heading? Periodontology 2000. 2017;73(1):241–58.

86. Wang W, Yeung KWK. Bone grafts and biomaterials substitutes for bone defect repair: a review. Bioactive Mater. 2017;2(4):224–47.

87. Thrivikraman G, Athirasala A, Twohig C, Boda SK, Bertassoni LE. Biomaterials for craniofacial bone regeneration. Dent Clin N Am. 2017;61:835–56.

88. Duminis T, Shahid S, Hill RG. Apatite glass-ceramics: a review. Front Mater. 2017;3:59.

89. Owen GR, Dard M, Larjava H. Hydroxyapatite/beta-tricalcium phosphate biphasic ceramics as regenerative material for the repair of complex bone defects. J Biomed Mater Res B. 2018;106:2493–512.

90. Bouler JM, Pilet P, Gauthier O, Verron E. Biphasic calcium phosphate ceramics for bone reconstruction: a review of biological response. Acta Biomater. 2017;53:1–12.

91. Dorozhkin SV. Biocomposites and hybrid biomaterials based on calcium orthophosphates. Biomatter. 2011;1(1):3–56.

92. Butz F, Bächle M, Ofer M, Marquardt K, Kohal RJ. Sinus augmentation with bovine hydroxyapatite/ synthetic peptide in a sodium hyaluronate carrier (PepGen P-15 Putty): a clinical investigation of different healing times. Int J Oral Maxillofac Implants. 2011;26(6):1317–23.

93. Dorati R, DeTrizio A, Modena T, Conti B, Benazzo F, Gastaldi G, et al. Biodegradable scaffolds for bone regeneration combined with drug-delivery systems in osteomyelitis therapy. In: Pharmaceuticals, vol. 10. Basel: MDPI AG; 2017.

94. Yang GH, Yeo M, Koo YW, Kim GH. 4D bioprinting: technological advances in biofabrication. In: Macromolecular bioscience, vol. 19. Weinheim: Wiley-VCH Verlag; 2019.

95. BioArchitects receives FDA approval for 3D printed titanium cranial plate. Available from: https://additivemanufacturingtoday.com/bioarchitects-receives-fda-approval-for-3d-printedtitanium-cranial-plate.

96. Srivastava, R., Tangade, P., & Priyadarshi, S. (2023). Transforming public health dentistry: Exploring the digital foothold for improved oral healthcare. *International Dental Journal of Students' Research*, *11*(2).

97. Srivastava, R., Tangade, P., Gahlaut, M. K., & Priyadarshi, S. SYSTEMATIC REVIEW OF THE RELATIONSHIP BETWEEN TOBACCO SMOKE AND CARBON MONOXIDE: IMPACT ON HEALTH AND DISEASE.

98. Srivastava, R., Tangade, P., Sahar, N., Priyadarshi, S., Pragya, A., & Ram, S. P. (2023). Scrutinizing paradigm between tooth wear facets and community's oral health: a review. *Eur Chem Bull*, *12*(4), 17848-55.

99. Srivastava, R., Tangade, P., Priyadarshi, S., Agarahari, P., & Kumari, T. (2023). The brewed connection: A comprehensive review of the relationship between caffeine and oral health. *International Journal of Dental Research*, *5*(2), 68-74.

100. Srivastava, R., Tangade, P., Singh, V., Priyadarshi, S., Dalai, S., Agarahari, P., ... & Singh, P. K. (2023). Chewing Ability and the Quality of Life: A Cross-Sectional Study to Assess the Relationship Between Tooth Wear and Oral Health. *Cureus*, *15*(7).

101. Srivastava, R., Tangade, P., Priyadarshi, S., Yadav, J., Pandey, H., & Kumar, V. M. S. (2023). Phytodentistry-An Obscure Yet Efficient Practise: A Review. *Int J Recent Sci Res*, *14*(5), 3073-6.

102. Srivastava, R., Tangade, P., Priyadarshi, S., Agarahari, P., Kumari, T., & Kumar, V. M. S. (2023). Protect your smile and your wallet: A review on dental insurance in India. *International Journal of Applied Dental Sciences, 9*(2), 271-275.

103. Agarahari, P., Jain, A., Tangade, P., Srivastava, R., Kumari, T., & Subhangi, S. (2023). Teledentistry: Transforming Dental Care Delivery and Education in the Digital Age. *Int J Dent Med Sci Res, 5*(3), 581-6.

104. Agarahari, P., Jain, A., Pandey, S. M., Agrahari, A. K., Yadav, J., Srivastava, R., ... & Sharma, Y. (2023). Exploring the Synergistic Association Between Oral Health Status and Oral Health Literacy Among College Students: A Cross-Sectional Study. *Cureus, 15*(7).

105. Srivastava, R., Tangade, P., Singh, V., Jain, A., Agarahari, P., & Pandey, H. (2022). Dental Informatics: Current Challenges and Opportunities For Providing Advanced Care In Dentistry. *TMU J Dent, 9*(3), 14-21.

106. Pandey, H., Tangade, P., Singh, V., Jain, A., Srivastava, R., & Sharma, M. (2024). To Correlate the Oral Health-related Quality of Life Between Smokers and Smokeless Tobacco Users Among 35–44 Years Age Group Attending Teerthanker Mahaveer Dental College and Research Centre, Moradabad, Uttar Pradesh, India. *Journal of Indian Association of Public Health Dentistry, 22*(2), 163-168.

107. Priyadarshi, S., & Srivastava, R. Unraveling the genetic basis of dental diseases: A comprehensive review.

108. Priyadarshi, S., Tangade, P., Sahar, N., & Srivastava, R. (2022). The Dermatoglyphics: Deciphering Dental Diseases. *University Journal of Dental Sciences, 8*(1).

109. Yadav, D., Jaiswal, P., Kumari, N., Jemini, I., Verma, Y., Tandon, S., & Srivastava, R. (2024). Knowledge, attitude, and practice regarding artificial intelligence (ai) and its usage in dental academics curriculum among dental undergraduates and postgraduates. *patient care, 1*, 2.

110. Srivastava, R., & Priyadarshi, S. (2024). Eyes on the future: Navigating dentistry's revolution with eye tracking technology. *International Dental Journal of Students' Research, 12*(2).

111. Jaggi, P., Priyadarshi, S., Gautam, J., Agarwal, N., & Srivastava, R. (2023). Artificial intelligence in dentistry: A boon or bane?. *Journal of Dental Specialities, 11*(2).

112. Agarahari, P., Jain, A., Tangade, P., Yadav, J., Srivastava, R., & Kumari, T. (2023). Topical fluorides: Fight against caries.

113. Gahlaut, M. K., Tangade, P., Singh, V., Jain, A., & Srivastava, R. (2023). Tobacco Control and Prevention in India. *Dent, 10*(3), 34-38.

114. Srivastava, R., Tangade, P., & Priyadarshi, S. (2023). Managing dental fluorosis: A guide to improving appearance of the teeth. *Archives of Dental Research, 13*(1), 25-29.

115. Yadav, J., Tangade, P., Jain, A., Singh, V., Singh, A. K., & Srivastava, R. (2021). A COMPLETE ASSESSMENT OF THE LITERATURE ON-COVID-19 AND DENTISTRY.

116. Srivastava, R., & Priyadarshi, S. Glimpsing beyond the glitter: Navigating the depths of oral piercings.

117. Yadav, J., Tangade, P., Jain, A., Pandit, S., & Srivastava, R. (2021). COVID-19 IMPACTS OF INTERVENTION AND RISK EXODUS PLAN FOR COMPETENT PEOPLE IN THE FIELD OF DENTISTRY.

118. Bhatia, D., Aman, S., Shivam, D. S. T., & Srivastava, R. ROLE OF PROBIOTICS IN DENTISTRY: A QUESTIONNAIRE BASED STUDY.

119. Pandey, H., Tangade, P., Singh, V., Jain, A., & Srivastava, R. To assess the awareness of tomato flu amongst post graduate students of Teerthankar Mahaveer Dental College and Research Centre Moradabad Uttar Pradesh.

120. Agarahari, P., Jain, A., Tangade, P., Singh, V., & Srivastava, R. Addressing the challenges and opportunities of dental auxiliaries: A review.

121. Kumari, T., Tangade, P., Singh, V., Jain, A., & Srivastava, R. Efficacy of Triphala extract, Manuka honey, and Chlorhexidine Mouthrinse against Plaque Accumulation and Gingival Inflammation among Undergraduates:-A Randomized Controlled Trial.

122. Dubey, D., Priyadarshi, S., & Srivastava, R. Medicinal plants in dentistry-A brief review.

123. Agarahari, P., Jain, A., Tangade, P., Singh, V., Yadav, J., & Srivastava, R. A Prospective Study Regarding Assessment of Knowledge Attitude and Practice among School going Children and the Impact of Oral Health Education on them.

124. Priyadarshi, S., Tangade, P., Sahar, N., & Srivastava, R. The COVID-19 delta or detrimental variant?.

125. Priyadarshi, S., Sahar, N., Srivastava, R., & Subhangi, S. Perceptions Regarding Covid-19 Vaccines Among General Population Visiting Tertiary Care Hospital in Moradabad, Uttar Pradesh.

126. Kumari, K., Solanki, P., Yadav, J., Gaur, A., Tandon, S., & Srivastava, R. KNOWLEDGE, ATTITUDE AND PRACTICE AMONG DIFFERENT DENTISTS REGARDING ORAL PIERCING DELETERIOUS EFFECT: A QUESTIONNAIRE BASED STUDY.

127. Agarwal, N., Priyadarshi, S., Jaggi, P., & Srivastava, R. Robotics in dentistry: Heading towards techno-verse era.

128. Agarahari, P., Tangade, P., Singh, V., Jain, A., Srivastava, R., & Pandey, H. ETHICS IN DENTISTRY.

129. Srivastava, R. (2023). *Correlation Between Teeth Wear and Oral Health Related Quality of Life Among Adult Patients*. GRIN Verlag.

130. Priyadarshi, D. S., Tangade, D. P., & Najm, D. dream for one and all.", 2021. *International Journal of Current Research*.